101 Tips for Surviving in a Pandemic

A Generation Z Guidebook

Kate Battaglia

Loving Healing Press
Ann Arbor, MI

ISBN 978-1-61599-645-2: paperback
ISBN 978-1-61599-646-9: hardcover
ISBN 978-1-61599-647-6: eBook

Audiobook available on iTunes and Audible.com

Published by
Loving Healing Press
5145 Pontiac Trail
Ann Arbor, MI 48105

www.LHPress.com
info@LHPress.com

Distributed by Ingram (USA/CAN/AU), Bertram's Books
(UK/EU)

This book is dedicated to those who
have lost their lives or loved ones to
COVID-19.

Contents

Introduction

During the past two years, COVID-19 has taken much from younger generations such as mine, restricting the ability of the young to socialize, compete in sports, work, and learn—our general education has been at risk. My name is Kate Battaglia, and I am currently a high schooler within the Dallas area. As a teen who has lived in Massachusetts, Montana, and currently Texas, my friendships are broad, and I am well aware of my generation's trials during a pandemic; the years 2020 and beyond will not be forgotten by any of us. My generation is called "Gen Z" or those born on or after the year 2000. We "zoomers" are not the baby boomers born earlier than 1964; we are not Gen X born from 1965-1980. We differ from the millennials born between 1981 and 1999. Gen Z is at the beginning of life choices and careers—and we are feeling the confusion and stress of COVID-19 at a time when baby boomers are retiring or retired (Harlow, 2021).

During the peak of the pandemic in the Spring of 2020, all the resources which had been available to the young such as restaurants, clothing stores, bookstores and particularly classrooms were brought to an abrupt cessation. The infamous heat and high temperatures that characterize the climate of the State of Texas were nowhere to be found within the desolate month of March, 2020. Our atmosphere was now characterized by a cool gray veneer and stray gusts of icy wind, which wove its way into the folds of our jackets. As restrictions tightened and tension rose surrounding the virus, adolescents like me were forced to endure quarantines, virtual classes, isolation, and eventually the option to take vaccines—which I did. My generation had to cultivate safe activities to keep us entertained for the months following the Spring of 2020. Although many people worry about our generation's stressors, studies do show "resilience or even possible benefits as a result of the lockdown...increased levels of perspective-taking and vigor, decreased levels of tension, and high levels of giving..." (van de Groep et al., 2021).

Clearly, I was blessed to have a personal computer, as streaming services such as Netflix, Hulu, and Disney+ gained great popularity while my friends and I spent increasing hours inside the confines of our homes—usually our bedrooms. As computer applications such as Zoom and Google Meet came to fruition, younger generations now had ways to spend digital movie nights with friends, play online games, or even hold book clubs. Vast numbers of people could all flood onto a single call with a mere copy and pasting of a link onto a group chat or other form of social media. Perhaps surprisingly, we each experienced our own individual personal growth throughout this past year as we spent more and more time with ourselves, yielding what seems to be a hint of increased maturity along with creativity.

Despite the great deal of innovation produced at the hands of young adults (as creative writing, computer game creation), today's Gen Zers mustn't forget the hardships we all collectively faced within this 2020-2021+ period. Personally, the strife I faced during this epidemic was largely overcome by the company and aid of my friends and family. In the face of future pandemics and widespread illness, we zoomers must do our best to remember how we overcame our collective hardships as a community, and as struggling individuals. The following 101 Tips are for you, the young of COVID-19 America!

.

101 Tips

1. **Find safe ways to connect**

   Before COVID-19, many Gen Zers took advantage of resources such as Zoom, group FaceTimes, and Google Meet. During the worst of the pandemic, with social media available, we were able to continue to have group movie nights, virtual parties, and other activities we would normally do in person. My favorite film was *Suspiria*!

2. **Socially distanced picnics**

   While picnics seem like the type of event parents might force teens to do with them on a humid summer afternoon, they are one of the best ways to connect with friends in a safe environment. Teens are in a time of "pulling away" from family and seeking time with peers; COVID-19 has interrupted our transition. My friends and I often have picnics at local parks or lakes.

3. **Bike rides**

   This could simply be hopping on your bike and pedaling through your neighborhood for a couple of minutes. Sometimes it's nice to take a break from the confines of your home and remind yourself of the bustling world outside. It's also a great way to rest your eyes from the extensive time they've been blankly staring at screens, either for school or for fun.

4. **Baking**

   Explore the depths of Google or maybe that cookbook that's been sitting on your shelf for the past year, unopened. Test out new recipes, or experiment. Now is a perfect time for cooking and eating healthy! Guys, you should learn to cook too! You could make a birthday cake for a friend—but don't make too much of a mess! I myself am not a talented baker and have made quite a few mistakes experimenting with new recipes. Remember to turn off the stove!

5. **Make new playlists**

   Pandemics provide us with an extensive amount of extra time to do as we please; listen to new music artists, experiment with different sounds, and group favorite songs together.

6. **Watch and review movies**

   Watch new movies, either popular or unheard of, and rate them like a critic would on the website *Rotten Tomatoes* (see www.rottentomatoes.com). Create a journal of all your responses, similar to a movie database. Whenever I finish watching a movie, I record my opinions and reactions in an app called Letterboxd. The app itself allows for you and your friends to see what you've watched and what you're planning to watch.

7. **Read!**

   As a junior in high school, I rarely get time to sit down and crack open a book, so use the time you have to explore some new literature. Personally, I am not a huge fan of romance books, but during quarantine I found myself completely enraptured by Jane Austin's *Northanger Abbey*. Romance novels are truly not as bad as I thought they were.

8. **Organize**

   Organizing and reorganizing your room, closet, or bathroom is an easy and productive way to pass time. The satisfaction of a newly organized space is a reward certainly worth the time and effort.

9. **Reach out to new friends**

   The COVID-19 pandemic has forced us to isolate for the sake of our personal health and that of others, making weekend hangouts with close friends a strenuous task to take on. Along with keeping in touch with old friends, try to reach out to others. Make new connections. Someone out there may need you! Connecting doesn't have to be digital; phone calls, texting and email are fine, but don't forget actual visits at safe distances, or even snail mail.

10. **Sit down and paint**

    Whether you consider yourself to be a skilled artist or not, sometimes it's fun to test your creativity on a blank canvas. Supplies such as watercolor, oil-based paint, pastels, and acrylic paint can be found at local craft stores or even CVS. My sister and I attempted to sketch with crayons; we did portraits of our grandparents. I think mine was surprisingly good, and maybe I'll take an art class in the near future.

11. Decorate old shoes

Recently I took up the project of redecorating my much-worn Nike Air Force 1s. All you need is acrylic paint, markers or pens, and an idea to run with (no pun intended)!

12. Meditate

A prominent issue facing younger generations during this pandemic is the mental stigma around self-isolation, often for safety. Apps that I personally use are Calm App and Headspace, which are both great resources for grounding and mindfulness. For any Harry Styles fans, the Calm App has a sleep story narrated by him.

13. Go on walks

After long days of staring at computer screens, a brisk stroll under a canopy of trees is just what our eyes need to relax. One of my favorite things to do is to grab some earbuds and listen to new bands or artists' music while I walk. When I bring my phone along on walks, I make sure to put it on "Do Not Disturb" or "Silent Mode" so I don't get distracted by any notifications. Janssen & Carradini (2021) report that Gen Z has "awareness of the negatives of technology use."

14. Buy chalk

Similar to painting, chalk drawing provides you with the infinite canvas of the outdoors. Walking around town or your neighborhood becomes a creative expedition where you can (literally) leave your mark on the world. Remember to research if it is legal to do so in the areas you choose to draw on.

15. **Test out new styles**

On a daily basis, we are exposed to varying styles through the mode of social media or even public observation. Test out any new styles that pique your interest. Society today (thankfully) welcomes a multitude of deviations in styles or "looks." Recently I've borrowed a lot of my dad's old jeans and vintage band t-shirts: use your resources!

16. **Try on new makeup looks**

Experiment with your eye shadow palette and other products and discover new looks as well as testing your own skills with a brush. Guys, there are products for you too! My male cousin just discovered the joys of hair gel.

17. **Seasonal activities with friends**

During quarantine last fall, a couple of friends and I made lists of "fall" or "winter" activities (depending on the season) to complete as a group. Last winter, my friends and I made holiday activities for each day until Christmas: these activities included watching Christmas movies over Zoom, holiday themed drawing contests, and making holiday playlists together.

18. **Take up gardening**

Plant an assortment of flowers for a vibrant décor, or even vegetables as a source of homegrown produce. Turn your windows into gardens using hanging baskets and planters, especially if you live in an apartment or simply don't have a yard.

19. **COVID Pups**

In my neighborhood, several young people have gone to animal shelters and adopted "COVID pups." It is a joy to see so many new canines walking around local streets—they look so happy that their joy is contagious. If dogs aren't up your alley, adopt a kitten if you will. Remember though, adopting a pet is a permanent responsibility. Treat your pet as though it is your own child.

20. Keep a journal

Try writing about your daily routine or specific events that made your day. Writing is a great way to release any jarred-up emotions from past hours or even days. You could even write about dreams from previous nights!

21. Reflect on your mental health

During extensive periods of isolation, it's quite common and to say the least, natural, for your mental health to decline to some extent. Take time to breathe. Evaluate your mood and where you are, mentally. Remember that it's OK to not always feel OK! Bana & Sarfarfaz (2020) discuss the "mental health ailments'' caused by COVID-19, so Gen Z needs to battle a tendency to succumb to stress.

22. Online worship

For churchgoers wary of a return to their place of worship, YouTube and Christian TV networks stream daily religious services free of charge.

23. Try Ancestry.com to trace your family history

Discover where your roots lie by looking into your family's past. Who knows, you could be a part of a line of royal blood! Recently I found out that I'm the third Kate Paris in my bloodline; I've told my friends to call me Kate Paris III from now on!

24. If unvaccinated for COVID

Use internet sources to stay current with vaccine developments and protocols. The World Health Organization and the FDA allow you to become more familiar with medicinal options. As of late December 2021, "at least 243,527,564 people, or 74% of the USA population have received at least one dose. Overall, 205,811,394 people or 63% of the population have been fully vaccinated" (see www.LHPress.com/genz). As of December 2021, Comirnaty and Pfizer-BioNTech, Moderna, and Janssen are all vaccines either approved by the FDA or "authorized for emergency use." (also on www.LHPress.com/genz). I've had two Pfizer shots; my grandparents have used Moderna and grandfather Robert even had his booster— grandmother Carolyn had COVID mildly 9/21 so she is waiting for an antibody test to see if a booster is needed for her. A debate is now raging in the USA—does the government have the right to order vaccines for its employees? Private company employees? Can federal law interfere with state legislation? The answers are not clear—or easy! My mother tracks our Texas county statistics on her phone each day, which I feel is an excellent idea for anyone.

25. Learn about earlier pandemics and what stopped them cold

Typhoid, measles, mumps, polio, smallpox—how have vaccines kept Gen Z from contracting these diseases? What is the MMR vaccine? You need to know how lucky Americans are to have been inoculated for measles, mumps, and rubella

(German Measles or 3-day Measles) [spend a little time on CDC.gov].

26. **Stay updated on COVID 19 variants**

Several good apps are free and can keep you up to date on the latest COVID-related news. Some of these are NHS COVID-19, HEALTHLYNKED COVID-19, and BetterHelp.

27. **Imagine your future**

Think of five or six possible jobs/professions you might like: Talk to people in those fields, research them, and possibly shadow them.

28. **Online shopping**

Find your favorite stores and ask friends for theirs. Which shops have easy returns? Which are the most reliable? Importantly, which local stores need your business in order to stay afloat? I personally like to shop at Aritzia, a clothing shop.

29. **Volunteer**

My mother and I have, with others, supported a school in North Dallas by finding out what supplies the school needs, and then helping to provide them. Contact UnitedWay.org for ideas about where and what to do.

30. **Forgive!**

Call or write to those who have hurt you in some way. If you live with such a person, talk it out—find a way to live a better life without hatred and guilt. As Malachy McCourt once said, "Resentment is like taking poison and waiting for the other person to die."

31. Confront the issue of masks

Find out what restaurants, museums, and shops are open in your area—wear a mask if mandated; at present the N95 mask seems safest. However if masks are not readily available to you, I do know people recycling old neckties and tees as they make personalized masks, and some have created a small business selling them. John Hopkins Medicine has clear instructions for how to make a masks. (see www.LHPress.com/genz)

32. Renew old acquaintances

I try, at least once every few days to call someone I've lost touch with and simply ask them about their lives.

33. Singing

Not all who play instruments can sing well. Those who do, like my sister Lauren, have managed to participate in local musical productions while wearing masks. Some shows have been videotaped and saved for a better day!

34. Take a break from social media

The more we linger on others' lives, the less we focus on ours. Live in the moment! Happiness is a daily decision. Spend at least one day, not merely a break, without social media, and record how this felt in your journal: Choudhary et al. (2021) conducted a webinar showing "More than half of the participants reported excessive social media engagement and screen time." It's hard not to be addicted to technology in a pandemic, but forming an addiction can be avoided with occasional days or hours out of doors.

35. Don't miss your prom

Surely there is a substitute! Meet up with a few good friends and hold your own COVID-safe prom/dance!

36. Redecorate your room

Hang posters, stack books, buy succulents (plants)! Print out pictures of friends or your top music artists and idols. I wish my parents would let me hang up posters, but they think I will damage the walls.

37. Dye your hair

A great introduction to a dramatic character change is different-colored hair. Add highlights or colored streaks. Maybe bleach your hair! Brunette guys can find out if blondes truly have more fun!

38. Write!

Pick up a pen and paper, and write your soul into your desired format, whether it be prose or poetry. Look up prompts or make your own. The best writing is produced when you're not afraid or worried about the reaction of others. Write for yourself. Experiment with new formats, spacing, or even writing styles.

39. Learn a new sport

Pick up a tennis racket or your parents' old bag of golf clubs—the options are limitless; some are indoor sports, like billiards or pool.

40. Knit!

While this may appear to be an activity only for your grandparents, there is much more to it than knitting a scarf or an ugly sweater. Knit your own cute tops, bags, or even blankets. Guys, did you see diver Tom Daley knitting at the Tokyo Olympics?

41. Go to an antique store

If it proves safe, go to your local antique store or mall, and browse around. Find hidden treasures and oddities that make you wonder "who would own something like this?"

42. Thrift!

Similar to antiquing, thrifting allows you to take a peek into others' lives through articles of clothing. Thrifting is an affordable way to find vintage pieces of clothing as well as supporting a local business. Art, furniture, and sports equipment are also excellent thrifting finds. I recently heard of a woman who found a strand of Mikimoto pearls in a Goodwill store in Virginia!

43. Support sustainable stores

Research which clothing stores you patronize are sustainable. Are they ethical? Do they benefit the environment? What do they support?

44. Start a book club

Grab a group of friends who enjoy reading, and pick the book of your choice. Analyze and discuss the book together. What do you like about it? Or dislike?

45. Learn how to make friendship bracelets

Get string from your local craft store and search the internet for designs. Ask friends if they know how to make bracelets, or even make bracelets for them! This small skill is not gender dependent.

46. Go to virtual concerts

Some music artists during the pandemic hold virtual concerts or listening sessions for their fans. Many of them are free of charge! I particularly enjoyed one by Billie Eilish.

47. Paint your nails

Try complicated designs, like checks or flowers. Try out new colors and styles: your nails can serve as an accent piece for your outfit. I wonder if my guy friends would let me paint their nails!

48. Learn how to make your own coffee or tea

Save money by making your own morning lattes, chai, or matcha.

49. Keep a schedule

Make a list of all your commitments with friends, school, doctors, or even personal goals. When pandemics rampage throughout our everyday lives, a schedule helps relieve us of stress as well as keeping us motivated to accomplish all planned tasks. You may find that using a calendar app is even better than a wall calendar.

50. Press flowers

While walking through your neighborhood, pick up any flowers or plants that catch your eye. Lay your collected plants between two sheets of paper, then press heavy books or magazines atop of your flowers. Wait a few weeks with the flowers under the books; then you'll achieve your final product of an assortment of frameable preserved plants. Guys, you can be the flower fetchers!

51. **Binge watch a Netflix/Hulu show**

    Over the COVID-19 pandemic, I watched count-
    less shows such as *Reign* or *Supernatural*. TV is
    another great way to pass time and wind down
    from daily stressors. Ask your friends for recom-
    mendations.

52. **Learn grounding exercises**

    The more time we have to ourselves, the more time
    we have to get lost within our minds. Remember to
    center yourself and recognize that you are in fact
    living in the present moment. You are not losing
    control, you are safe.

53. **Learn a different language**

    The internet provides you with endless amounts of
    resources free of cost. Websites such as YouTube,
    Duolingo, and Rosetta Stone are great resources.
    Many libraries are currently open, providing
    internet access free of charge. The sky's the limit!

54. **Buy scented candles**

    Set the mood and/or atmosphere of your room
    with the scent of your choice. Just remember to
    blow them out when you leave! (Guys, this beats
    the smell of sweaty socks, I promise.)

55. **Make your own candles**

    Websites such as YouTube and Pinterest as well as
    apps like TikTok can provide you with much of
    the information and tutorials you need. Bend the
    wax in odd shapes and make abstract designs.
    What scent are you going to use? Warning: Don't
    use pumpkin.

56. Buy a disposable camera

Carry it around with you at all times and capture the moments you wish to preserve on film. Out of personal experience, I believe the best pictures are taken at night or in the dark. Those lucky enough to have smartphones can use the cameras they already have.

57. Stop procrastinating!

Procrastination is arguably one of the greatest enemies of our generation. It devours our free time with an unquenchable thirst for empty minutes, and we must overcome its tyrannical reign by taking the initiative and knocking out homework or chores needing to be done as early as possible.

58. Make a sleep schedule

I can't emphasize how important sleep is for not only our physical health, but for mental health as well. Managing to get over 7 hours of sleep every day can reduce anxiety and stress held over from the previous day. Sometimes schoolwork can compromise your ability to get a healthy amount of rest, but remember to not make shirking homework a habit. With substantial sleep, your mind can work to its full potential. (see www.LHPress.com/genz)

59. Take naps!

While this may sound like a mindless task, naps are a great way to recover missed hours of sleep. Again, lack of sleep augments stress, so take naps as a form of de-stressing.

60. **Look through family picture or scrapbooks**

    Delve into your past with memorabilia held onto by either you or your parents. Relive your childhood memories or even uncover memories you didn't even know you had. Think of all the memories lost by tornado victims in Kentucky (12/21)—and treasure yours.

61. **Find a study group**

    Finding a group of people to study with acts as a motivator to complete upcoming assignments or projects. Talk about upcoming tests or go over work together. Don't get distracted too easily!

62. **If in need of mental and emotional support**

    Reach out to the crisis text line; text HOME to 741741, and/or if you need more support, please reach out to the National Suicide Prevention Hotline at 800-273-8255. Personal counseling can be costly or free; church pastors, rabbis, or priests can also be a wonderful resource.

63. **Build a support system**

    Even if you are in a stable place mentally, developing a group of people you can call when you fall into your lows is a great resource to have. REMEMBER THOUGH, always ask permission to vent to someone!

64. **Learn which demographics are impacted most in a time of pandemic**

    In a study of the effects of the pandemic on undergraduates, it was found that female students were ultimately more impacted mentally than male students. Female students who live in a household with insufficient income or lacking employment are found to have increased mental health ailments (Bana & Sarfaraz, 2020).

65. **Take an online class**

If you don't have time in your fractured school schedule to take Spanish (for example), take a beginner's course online. If you don't own your own computer or have internet access, go to any library that is still open.

66. **Gap semesters or years**

For those going off to college, realize that your campus rules may change in a heartbeat. If face-to-face classes become digital, or if dorms are closed, a gap term/year may be the answer. In the gap one can still find jobs like data entry online. For Gen Zers in college or not, Chick-fil-A is wide open for employment—as are myriad businesses.

67. **Get your endorphins pumping**

Despite the fact that a pandemic may isolate sports teams, you can still play sports outdoors— swimming, basketball, tennis, etc. There are so many activities you can do without money or access to a gym, such as walking, running, or free H-I-I-T workouts on YouTube.

68. **Subscribe to magazines or newspapers**

Stay up to date on the latest fashion trends in *GQ* and *Vogue*, or keep up to date with current events with *The New York Times*.

69. **Master software**

Schools across the nation are using different software programs to allow online classes; some have changed software multiple times. Learn to be more proficient at your school's chosen programs such as Schoology, Canvas, Microsoft Teams, etc.

70. **Start a club**

    Email your school's club organizers and give them your pitch! Get a group of interested friends and acquaintances and hold your own meetings. This is also a great way to add onto leadership roles for your work or college resume.

71. **Go out on a date**

    Whether it's romantic or platonic, find someone to go out with. Have a nice dinner at a COVID-safe restaurant, or even have a picnic.

72. **Apply for local jobs**

    Search on websites such as LinkedIn to find local job opportunities either in person or online. Earn your own money to buy whatever pleases you, or save up for something expensive.

73. **Go to an art gallery or museum**

    Take a peek into the past through art pieces and sculptures from centuries past. Find out what inspired artists of past years to produce their masterpieces.

74. **Buy Tarot cards**

    Find reliable resources online on how to use a deck as well as the meaning behind each card. Do readings for friends and family! You might enjoy *The True Nature of Tarot* by Diane Wing.

75. **Make a time capsule**

    Gen Z, how about making a time capsule featuring these pandemic years, and burying it somewhere special? I'd like to contribute a nasal swab!

Newspaper articles can show conflicting views from scientists and governments regarding the origin of COVID-19. Maybe those who dig up this capsule will already have found a simple and easy cure—I hope so!

76. **Learn how to play solitaire**

Solitaire is a great way to test your mental capabilities without the need of another player. This is yet another way to pass time while simultaneously exercising your mind! My favorite is clock solitaire.

77. **Learn how to do calligraphy**

This is a creative way to play with your own handwriting as well as to improve it. Write down the names of friends. Use vibrant colors! I watched a YouTube video called "How To: Calligraphy & Hand Lettering for Beginners! Tutorial + Tips!" by the channel called AmandaRachLee, which was fun and helpful (see www/LHPress.com/genz).

78. **Shop for senior neighbors**

Reach out to older neighbors and offer to run errands for them. Delivery services can be quite expensive, so this is a great way to save others money and help at-risk neighbors!

79. **Teach your pet a new trick**

Teach your dog how to bark on command or teach your bird how to sing a popular song!

80. **Learn to play an instrument**

Look up tutorials online or call up a friend who plays the instrument of your choice. This October I started to teach myself how to play the guitar, and now I can't put it down!

81. Start a band

This is for you if you have a passion for music. Call up friends who can sing or play the guitar. Perform for your classmates and other friends!

82. Learn sign language

Learn it with your friends! Have secret conversations with them from afar, and not to mention silently.

83. Learn Morse code

Communicate with others with the blink of an eye or a quiet pencil tap. Send secret messages to others without anyone noticing. When I was younger, my neighbor and I learned Morse code because we thought her cat was trying to communicate with us by tapping her tail!

84. Try sleeping with music

Getting lost in your thoughts? Find playlists with ambient noises or the rumble of thunder. Spotify is a great resource for this because of its sleep timer option. My favorite sleep playlist is called "Floating Through Space" on Spotify. (see www.LHPress.com/genz).

85. Get abs!

Use apps such as Nike Training Club to find workout routines to match your desires. Many isometric workouts don't require the use of any equipment, except an open space. Remember not to push yourself too hard. I occasionally forget to give myself rest days and I end up making myself sick, or worse than I felt before!

86. **Go on virtual college tours**

    As college applications approach, virtual tours are safe ways to become acquainted with any college/ university campus without leaving the confines of your home.

87. **Pick up litter**

    Walk around your neighborhood with a trash bag and gloves and pick up any wrappers or bottles strewn across the ground.

88. **Ask your parents or caretakers for old clothes**

    This is another sustainable way to find new clothes, but now free of cost. It is useful way to find vintage clothes and experiment with old styles.

89. **Manifest something**

    Find something you hope will happen, whether it's a feeling or event, and look online for techniques to use. Learn how to make sigils!

90. **Go see live music if possible**

    Dallas often has small popup performances— mainly outside—with smaller groups or local artists. See if your city or town has any socially-distanced live music events that would be safe and fun to attend.

91. **Build a LEGO structure**

    LEGOs were a significant part of my childhood, so my family and I still have bins teeming with LEGO bricks. Make a castle, or even a hospital of your own.

92. Perform a play

Have your family or friends act out a play, such as Shakespeare's *The Comedy of Errors* or even *Hamlet*. The world is your stage!

93. Vlog your daily routine

Use your phone or camera and record significant events throughout your day. Post it online or simply pretend you're a famous influencer. FYI, a vlog is a personal website for social media videos.

94. Donate to charities

If you lack safe ways to volunteer locally, find causes you support online, and donate!

95. Learn chess strategies

After watching *The Queen's Gambit* on Netflix, I developed the sudden urge to battle someone in the strategic game of chess. Research techniques online and test them out against others, and surprise them with your newfound capabilities! Did you know you can reach checkmate in two moves?

96. Go to a drive-in theater

With the pandemic at its peak, movie theaters shut down, forcing us to watch upcoming movies on the screens of our TVs. Drive-in movies can provide you with the same theater-like experience within safe measures.

97. Go on a road trip

Bring friends and family and drive to wherever your heart draws you. Drive to a beach or the mountains!

98. Call your grandparents

The pandemic made it unsafe for older relatives to come into contact with the young for lonely months. Make sure to stay connected during these times of isolation.

99. If you don't have computer access

If you know someone without a computer, or someone with a specific need, check out www.givingcenter.org and www.withcauses.org for ways to help.

100. Try going vegan

Change your diet and see how it makes you feel. Maybe you'll find a lifestyle worth sticking with. My family and I tried to go vegan for a short period of time, but my dad caved and made burgers the next night! Certain diets aren't for everyone I suppose.

101. Remember to love

Remind your parents, siblings, friends, relatives, as well as yourself that you love them. Sometimes we forget to show how much we care about others.

Afterword from Kate

As the COVID-19 virus continues to manifest variants like Delta and Omicron, more vaccines and treatments will probably emerge. Schools and workplaces may continue to leapfrog from digital to face-to-face and back to the digital realm. Gen Z is trying to find itself in the midst of a changing pandemic; therefore, Gen Z may be the source of original and worthy plans to maintain growth and sanity in a confusing and frightening world. Gen Z may also need help in dealing with stress and depression. I hope these tips get minds flowing into constructive places, because we simply do not know how and when the COVID-19 pandemic will end; we don't know if our schools or workplaces will be digital or face-to-face or a combination of both. As the Federal government and fifty state legislatures debate COVID-19 protocols, we can only hope their plans will coalesce...so good luck! KB

References

Bana, K. F., & Sarfaraz, S. (2020). Impact on Mental Health of Undergraduates and the Ways to Cope Stress during COVID-19 Pandemic. *Pakistan Armed Forces Medical Journal*, 70(5), 1453-1459.

Choudhary, S., Nebhinani, N., Arora, I. K., & Paul, K. (2021). Thriving through COVID-19: Promoting resilience in adolescents. *Journal of Indian Association for Child & Adolescent Mental Health*, 17(1), 142–145.

Harlow, J. (2021) Gen Z Is Facing Work-Life Struggles. *TD: Talent Development*, 75(6), 14-15.

Janssen, D., & Carradini, S. (2021). Generation Z Workplace Communication Habits and Expectations. *IEEE Transactions on Professional Communications* 64(2), 137-153.

van de Groep, S., Zanolie, K., Green, K. H., Sweijen, S. W., & Crone, E. A. (2020). A daily diary study on adolescents' mood, empathy, and prosocial behavior during the COVID-19 pandemic. *PLoS ONE*, 15(10), 1–20.

Index

About the Author

Kate Battaglia is 17 years old, born in 2004 in Boston, Massachusetts. She was raised in Wellesley, MA where she attended schools through the 6th grade. Her family then moved to Dallas, Texas, where Kate and her younger sister enrolled in a north Dallas school. During the early stages of the COVID-19 pandemic, Kate attended school digitally, later switching to face-to-face classrooms. Many of her peers contracted COVID; she herself had one false positive test, and later chose to be vaccinated. Kate loves her dog Fenway, enjoys a variety of sports (especially snow-skiing), and loves to write. She is ambitious, taking numerous Advanced Placement and Honors classes in this, her junior high school year. She has been published in her high school literary magazine, and won a grade-level school award for English. Spending summers in Montana, Kate has also been published in *Explore Big Sky*. In her *101 Tips for Surviving a Pandemic: A Generation Z Guidebook*, Kate speaks for Gen Z—those born near the year 2000. Her tips are at times surprising, showing readers how positive and creative Gen Zers can be.

CPSIA information can be obtained
at www.ICGtesting.com
Printed in the USA
BVHW011458310122
627620BV00001B/12

9 781615 996469